WATER

INFUSED

RECIPES

Water Infused Recipes For Natural Weight loss

Dr IRENE JACKSON

TABLE OF CONTENTS

16*Barked Pear With Sage Infusion

17*Mixed Melody Infusion

18*Blueberry Lime and Cilantro Infusion

19*Apple Orange and Raspberry Infusion

20* Berry Mingle Infusion

21*pepper and strawberry Infusion

22*Citrus Sensation Infusion

23*Cocumber and Lemon Infusion

24* and Grapefruit Infusion

25*Rosemary Berries and Vanilla Infusion

26*Refreshing Lime Strawberry Infusion

27* Fizzy Citrus Infusion

28*Day Spa Grapefruit Pineapple Infusion

29*Cayenne pepper and slices

30*Lemon and Pomegranate Infusion

31*Grape and Pineapple Infusion

32*Hibiscus and Exotic Mandarin Infusion

34*Berries Lime and Mint Infusion

34*Hibiscus and Star Fruit Orange

Infusion

35*Strawberry and Jalapeno Infusion

36*Berry Blast Infusion

37* Strawberry and Basil Infusion

38*Raspberry and Pineapple Infusion

39*Orange Infusion

40*Tropical Mango Infusion

INTRODUCTION

Thank you, and congratulations! Thank you

For obtaining the ebook Infused Water: 40 Infused

Vitamin Water Recipes For Natural Weight Loss, Detox,

and Healthy Living. I am privileged to guide you on this

quest to develop quick & easy infused water recipes!

Some people believe that water is too monotonous and

uninteresting to drink in large numbers, even though it is

essential for human health and existence. Others prefer

flavorful liquids, while some receive water from tea or

coffee. These liquids provide the hydration we require,

but they also significantly increase the sugar we

consume daily, which we know can have no health

effects .

BENEFITS

If you surveyed a wide range of people about their health behaviors, you would undoubtedly find that many do not consume enough water. This is a typical admission made by innumerable individuals who understand that the advantages of drinking water exceed the disadvantages of not drinking enough of it. Fortunately, a novel approach to drinking water has recently gained popularity and is sweeping the health community. Not only among dietitians and celebrities but also among the people concerned about their health, infused water is steadily rising in popularity. Simple ingredients like fruit or herbs are added to water to make it taste better. This practice is known as "infused water .

Ingredients for Orange-Papaya Agua Fresca

InChapterfused Water 4 cups ripe papayas, peeled, seeded, and cubed (about 3) 1 freshly squeezed orange juice, half a cup freshly squeezed lime juice, 1/4 cup 1.4 cups of water 2 tbsp. honey (optional) Crushed ice or ice cubes Orange segments, clementine segments, or slices Directions * Blend papayas, orange juice, and lime squeezed lime juice, 1/4 cup 1.4 cups of water 2 tbsp. honey (optional) Crushed ice or ice cubes Orange segments, clementine segments, or slices Directions * Blend papayas, orange juice, and lime .

CHAPTER 2

Ingredients for Pink Grapefruit and Strawberry Infused Water 1/2 a cucumber without seeds strawberries, one pint Pink grapefruit, 1 little Splenda 1 cup Peel the cucumber, reserving only a few narrow strips of the green peel. The strawberries should be hulled and cut crosswise into thin slices before being placed in a two quart pitcher. *Fill the pitcher with them. * Trim the grapefruit's ends. Cut into thick slices and then wedges. * Add the wedges to the pitcher along with the strawberries and cucumber. * Splenda should be dissolved in two cups of water. Pour into the pitcher, then top off with more water. *Place in the fridge for two to three hours. Serve with fruit garnish over ice.

Ingredients for Tarragon Blueberry and Raspberry Tang Infused Water Blueberries, strawberries, and tarragon leaves Directions for Water Pour roughly 1 cup of water to be at the bottom of a 2-to2 44-quart pitcher. Use a wooden spoon to lightly muddle the fruit and crush the leaves after adding the ingredients. Add water on top, then chill for at least one hour. Icing should be added soon before serving.

Ingredients for Ginger, Mint, and Lemon Infused Water depending on how strong you want your infused "water" to taste, 1-2 liters of filtered water; One ginger root, in part Piece of one lemon leaves of fresh mint (approx. 12-15) An ice cube (optional) The ginger root and lemons should be cut into slices, and the lemon back should be removed. Removing the fruit's skin off helps prevent Taking in some pesticides. * Jug with filtered water filled. Add lemon and ginger. Add a few fresh, mint leaves. You can also squeeze some lemon juice into the water to give it that nice of citrus flavor. The flavors will penetrate into the water if you let the mixture remain in the refrigerator all night. Daily pour, sip, and delight.

Things to use for infused water with mint and blueberries. 1.5 cups blueberries Mint, mixed, two sprigs two quarts of water Directions All the ingredients should be put in a jar and chilled to taste.

CHAPTER 6

Preparation for mix Herbs-Infused Water . basil leaves, 3 Rosemary, 1 little sprig Dill, two stalks one stem of lemon thyme or mint 30 oz. of water Fill a jar with water and put all the contents. Allow at least six hours to chill then serve .

CHAPTER 7

Ingredients for Tangelo Dream Infused Water 10 small cut of strawberries divided into 6 jars of cool clean filtered water 4 sprigs of fresh mint, nicely crushed, into two sliced tangelos, Fill the water to the bottom of a 2- to 2-quart pitcher about halfway with water. Add the mint and gently mash the leaves with a spoon made of wood. Add the strawberry and tangelo then later add the remaining water. Let the food rest for at least one hour. Just before serving, add some cubes of ice made of clean filtered water.

Water With a Savory Cucumber Flavor Ingredients: 20 slices of cucumber, divided into 6 jars of cool clean filtered water. two thinly cut lemons 4 fresh thyme sprigs, nicely crushed 2 fresh rosemary sprigs, nicely crushed Fill the jar to bottom of a 2- to 2-quart pitcher with about 1 cup of water. Add the thyme and rosemary, then lightly mash the herbs with a spoon made of wood or muddler. Add the lemon and cucumber then pour in the remaining water. Let the food rest for at least one hour. Just before serving, add cubes of ice produced with a clean filtered water.

Ingredients for Water With Strawberry Kiwi Bliss 9 ripe strawberries 1 kiwi 8 glasses of filtered or bottled water Washing, removing the leaves, and slicing in half are the instructions for strawberries. Kiwi should be washed, peeled, and cut. Water, strawberries, and kiwis are added in a 244-quart pitcher. Placing the container in the refrigerator should be done with care. A piece of wrap should be placed on over the top of a jar pitcher with no lid.

Ingredients for Water with Apple Pie Flavor 1 nicely sliced delicious apple, preferably a Fuji. 2 cinnamon sticks (make sure the powder on is not used it wouldn't dissolve) Directions the teapot approach Place all the ingredients in the teapot. Cover with water and bring to a boil. Serve in a tea cup or travel mug and, you can add additional cinnamon stick and stir . the teacup approach Add 1/4 of your apple slices and 1/2 of a cinnamon stick to a tea cup or travel mug. Pure hot water on the apples and cinnamon stick. allow it 2-4 minutes to cool down before you drink. Fill the tea cup with hot water until the flavor is no more .

CHAPTER 11

Ingredients for Orange-Pineapple and Ginger Infused Water 1/2 cup of orange cubes   sliced Pineapple in half Fresh grated ginger, 1 tablespoon quart-sized jars Wooden Spoon, Water, and Agave or another sweetness (optional) Directions

Put the ingredients in the glass jar to the bottom .Use a wooden spoon to stir.Put water in the jar.

Enjoy as is or chill overnight for the best flavor.

CHAPTER 12

Ginger- and Mango-Infused Water

Ingredients ginger root, 1 inch, peeled and sliced

Directions 1 cup Frozen Mango-Fresh one .

Use a spoon handle or a peeler to peel the ginger.

Only the portion you will be utilizing should be peeled.

 Cut the ginger into three to four slices the size of coins.Drop the mango into the jar then. Put some water, then add 3 cube of Ice

Place in refrigerator one to three hours before serving.

 When serving, place a few frozen mango pieces into the ice glass.

Mango Ginger Water can be stored in the refrigerator for 24 hours in cube form.

CHAPTER 13

Ingredients for Veggie Combo Infused Water Cucumber slices Carrot slices Celery slices Sweet or Hot peppers remove the seed and diced .Add Water as needed Directions Combine all ingredients in a jar of water. Relax   and drink

CHAPTER 14

Mandarin, Black Tea, and Basil leave Infused Water
Ingredients 4 piece of mandarin oranges, 5 basil leaves,
and 1 black tea bag Directions Combine all ingredients in
a jar. Add water on top. Maintain at room temperature
for two to three hours. Serve with ice.

CHAPTER 15

Ingredients for the preparation of Sage-Infused Water with Barked Pear About 20 ounces of water 2 to 3 slices of pear, cinnamon sage bud To taste, honey (If using , use a clean Plates for the raw honey) Instructions Add the fruit, the spices, and honey (if using) to an oven and bake for about 25 minutes at 350°F to infuse. Before taking it, give the food at least some minutes to cool in the refrigerator.

CHAPTER 16

Ingredients for the Traditional Cocumber and mint Infused Water Sliced cucumber with mint leaves that have been shredded and lightly crushed in the hand Water Instructions Combine all the ingredients in a jar. As desired, then serve chilled.

CHAPTER 17

Mixed Melodies with water . Ingredients One cucumber slice and one tangerine one grapefruit 3mint leaves, please liquids. Directions Combine all the ingredients in a jar, then serve it all day long.

Ingredients for Preparing Cilantro, Lime, and Blueberry Infused Water Little blueberries Fresh Cilantro Stalk two cut limes Directions for Water Combine all the ingredients in a container. Mix gently, then chill and serve.

Ingredients for Preparing Orange,Apple Water Infused and Raspberry Sliced, 12 apple, cut, and a cup of red raspberries. 24 ounces of water Instructions: Put the fruit in a mason jar . Close it after adding some water. Leave for like 30 minutes or overnight in the refrigerator. Then Serve.

CHAPTER 20

Components of infused water with lemon and pomegranate. Pomegranate seeds in a small amount 20 Lemons, 2 slices 8-9 ounces of water For the pomegranate juices to come out, gently smash the seed. Set inside the jar with the lemons. Add some water to the top. 4 hours of cooling. Serve after straining.

CHAPTER 21

Ingredients for preparing Water Flavored with Pepper and Strawberry   4 strawberries a pepper jar of water Cut strawberries in half after removing the tops. Thumb within plastic wrap or a glove, remove seeds from pepper. Add to the water-filled jar. For about 4–13 hours, cover and place in the fridge .

CHAPTER 22

Ingredients for preparing Citrus Sensation Infused Water 2 sliced lemons, and 13 piece of cucumber ,12 leaves of mint 4 gallons of water Directions Combine all of the ingredients together. Drink it warm after letting it steep all night

CHAPTER 23

Ingredients for preparing Cucumber and Lemon Infused Water 2 slices of natural lemon three slices of fresh cucumber 8 to 10 ounces of filtered water Put the lemon and the cucumber in a container. Sprinkle the ingredients with water. nighttime departure Drink when you first wake up in the morning.

CHAPTER 24

Ingredients for Preparing Rosemary and Grapefruit Infused Water 1 grapefruit 1 rosemary sprig 32 oz. Cut the grapefruit into slices after removing the rind. Fill the jar with water. Submerge the fruit and then add the rosemary. Keep for about 24 hours in the Refrigerator or two more hours at room temperature.

Ingredients for Preparing Water Infused with vanilla, Berries, and Rosemary Water, pure, 26 ounces 2 cups lightly mushed, seedless berries one or two entire vanilla beans Rosemary, 3 to 5 sprigs ,A tea spoon. The ingredients should be added to the bottle after opening the infuser. Pour water on it, and add cube ice if desired. ° Snap the lid on the infuser bottle. For the mixture to mix properly combine all and shake. Maintain for at least 3hours and Serve

CHAPTER 26

Ingredients for Preparing Refreshing Water With Strawberry and Lime . Infuse about 8 fresh strawberries 1 Lime 2 liters of Pellegrino or Club Soda, or plain water The strawberries should be cut into three parts. Put your feet in the water. Ten lime wedges should be cut and added to the water. After 3–4 hours of chilling, serve.

CHAPTER 27

Ingredients in Fizzy Citrus Infused Water Orange, Lemon, and Lime Clean water or flavor-infused soda water Instructions .Slice the lime and lemon, then give them a light squeeze. Put inside jar. Add water on top, then chill for at least one hour. When nicely cooled, serve.

Day Spa Apple, Pineapple, and Grapefruit Infused Water

.Ingredients Grapefruit, Half 1/2 Apple

Fresh Ice and Water with a Half of a Pineapple

Directions Grapefruit and Apple should be sliced into medium-sized pieces. Add to an attractive juice pitcher.Slice the pineapple into medium-thick or thinner pieces. Make every slice as uniformly sized as possible.If you want it more sweeter then squeeze some pineapple juice to give it a very sweet taste.

Add two cups of ice, then pour water on top of that.

Keep in the refrigerator for four hours

cayenne pepper in infuse water and peach slices

Cut slices of fresh peaches of . Cayenne pepper.

Instructions Place in water-filled jar. Stir and chill as you

Desire.

CHAPTER 30

Ingredients for Preparing Mingle Berry Infused Water, 3 cups of mixed blueberries and 12 strawberries, sliced 2 gallons of water Place the berries in a container as directed. The water should be added. Stir, then serve.

Ingredients for Preparing the Water With Berry Blast 1 cup of blueberries a cup of blackberries 1 2/2 cups pomegranate seeds 2-quarts of water Directions Pomegranate seeds should be frozen on ice trays. Blackberry and Blueberries can be cut into slices. soak in the water for about 5 hours Enjoy your drink when added the pomegranate seed cubes ice .

CHAPTER 32

Ingredients for preparing Hibiscus and Exotic Mandarin Infused Water 3 and half-cut mandarin oranges. 1 tablespoon of hibiscus blossoms Water or 1 tea bag , 32 ounces Put the items in a jar as directed. Add water to the top of the jar. Place in the fridge for 4-6 hours. Use a metal strainer to filter then serve chill

Ingredients for preparing Infused Water with Lime, Berries, and Mint Oranges, 1/8 cup 2 lime slices Mint, two sprigs A lemon slice, two basil sprigs, and three strawberries. 2 cucumber slices, some blueberries, a strawberry, and some mint. Flow Directions The components should be put in a jar. Mash the ingredients just a bit. Add water and ice to the top.

Serve after allowing it to chill for a few hours.

Ingredients for preparing infused water with orange ,star fruit, and hibiscus 2 teaspoons of loose hibiscus tea, or two teabags a sliced organic orange, three 4 slices of star fruit 80 oz. Put in a jar center, add the orange and tea together .Put water to fill the jar. Star fruit should be added. 6–14 hours are needed to chill then serve

CHAPTER 35

Chaptand Strawberries Infused Water 5 organic strawberries, a jalapeño pepper, and 35 ounces of water are combined. Directions Strawberries and jalapenos should be put in a jar. Over the ingredients, pour water. Cover and properly chill

Ingredients for Preparing Jalapeno

Ingredients for Preparing the Water With Berry Blast 1 cup of blueberries a cup of blackberries 1 2/2 cups pomegranate seeds 2-quarts of water Directions Pomegranate seeds should be frozen on ice trays. Blackberry and Blueberries can be cut into slices. soak in the water for about 5 hours Enjoy your drink when added the pomegranate seed cubes ice .

Ingredients for Preparing Strawberry and Basil Infused Water 12 strawberries, 5 basil leaves, quartered tom, and 3 quarts of water were blended. Place the ingredients in a container as directed. Before serving, cover and chill.

CHAPTER 38

Ingredients for preparing water infused with Pineapple and Raspberries. Several raspberries and pineapples 10–12 oz. of water Directions put a big glass with all the ingredients. Blend gently. Add water to the top. Well chilled, then serve.

Ingredients for preparing water infused with Pineapple and Raspberries. Several raspberries and pineapples 10–12 oz. of water Direction Fill a big glass with all the ingredients. Blend gently. Add water to the top. Well chilled, then serve.

Ingredients for preparing infused water with orange ,star fruit, and hibiscus 2 teaspoons of loose hibiscus tea, or two teabags a sliced organic orange, three 4 slices of star fruit 80 oz. Put in a jar center, add the orange and tea together .Put water to fill the jar. Star fruit should be added. 6–14 hours are needed to chill.then serve .

Who the Author Is

IRENE JACKSON is a writer of books on nutrition and weight loss. Her goal is to assist people in achieving their weight loss objective.She is respected in the wellness and fitness industry.

IRENE JACKSON has devoted her time to inspiring, motivating, and educating individuals to adopt positive philosophies and lifestyles.

As a trainer, she began her fitness career. She discovered that people must achieve their objectives and have the proper attitude.

Irene enjoys cooking nutritious meals, reading, exercising, and trying out new diet recipes in her free time.California is where Irene is now residing. As a

Health and Fitness Writer, she is employed. She adores....